One Hundred Calorie Appetite

Combined
With The

Five Minute
Workout ©

**Eat all day, every day.
Work out in five minute increments.
Never be hungry and feel the fat melt away.**

Josey Klearley

Dedication

**Whether you are a king or a pawn
playing in the game of life,
when the game is finished
we all wind up in the same box.**

**Regardless of how you played the game,
after all your time is spent as a pawn,
did you ever know the King of Kings?**

**A philosophical and practical approach
to healthy eating, exercising and living.**

*This book is dedicated to my mother Nancy.
She was a nutrition specialist for our hospital,
and a specialist in the development of my heart.*

*My special thanks to my wife Trudy for her
inspiration. Along with her love, support and help
she encouraged me to share what I've learned.*

The One Hundred Calorie Appetite With The Five Minute Workout

Eat all day long. Work out in five minute increments.
Never be hungry and feel the fat melt away.

A booklet and outline suggesting eating habits and cardio exercises.
Five days of eating: Five days of five minute workouts: Two days off.
Quick and easy recipes for snacks and shakes provided for the two days off.

Forward:

It's no accident that you chose to spend time to read this. Most likely, at this juncture, you have nothing invested - no time, no effort and no money. Therefore, take it for what it is worth and what it has cost you so far. This booklet is intended to be a gift given to you by someone who genuinely cares about you, your health, and your future. If you find it helpful and it helps accomplish your goal, then we ask you to please "pay it forward." Give this copy away to another person and help make an investment in someone else's life.

I want to share what I am not, and what I am. I have no medical training, and I am not a physician. I am not a nutrition specialist. I am not a behavioral scientist, nor am I a physical trainer. I am however, a middle aged, overweight, heart patient with a hypo-thyroid and partially torn rotator cuff. I needed to find a different way to lose my weight with minimal pain and effort as possible!

Obesity, diabetes and heart disease are some of the leading health problems facing our nation. My Grandmother died of complications from diabetes. My Uncle Ed died from a heart attack in his early fifties. My mother has had three separate angioplasties and stints. My father had heart disease and his first open heart surgery when he was thirty seven. In his fifties he had triple bypass surgery, and in his sixties he had several heart stints. When he passed away of natural causes, the only blood flow to his heart was the collateral blood vessels the heart grew to supply blood to the muscle because the arteries were 100% blocked. Our families' genetic history precluded that I needed to be acutely aware of my health.

In November of 2007 I was forty-eight years old, and I had a ladder slip out from under me. I fell and broke my right humorous arm bone and partially tore my rotator cuff. I share this with you because it directly affects and limits any upper body exercises and use of my arm. I have difficulty with swimming activities, basketball playing, racquetball activities, or lifting weights. Ironically, the damage to my rotator cuff actually helped my golf game. It forced me to slow my swing down and I hit the ball better than ever before! My wife now encourages me to golf because I can use the extra walking to get good exercise for at least nine holes without feeling guilty about playing!

During my forty ninth year of age, I lost forty pounds in twelve months by eating all day, every day, with no additional exercise. I took advice from a friend and I ate one hundred calories every hour on the hour. I lost weight naturally by using my body's metabolism and allowing my body to do the work on my behalf.

Twelve months into my new eating habit, and forty pounds lighter, I had a heart attack at age fifty. It took three angioplasty balloons and one stint to clear the blockages. I immediately quit smoking a pack a day, but over the next two years I had gained back fifty-two pounds. When walking, I was easily winded. I had trouble bending over to pick up a pen off the floor. My knees, ankles, and hips hurt. My sister is a physician's assistant for an orthopedic surgeon and warned me that I could be facing knee and hip replacement if I didn't lose my extra weight. At my last physical, my doctor told me I "needed to diet, exercise, and lose weight." It was easy for him to say, just very difficult for me to do. What he didn't tell me is what I want to tell you. I discovered that I could eat all day long, work out in only five minute increments, and let my body melt away the extra fat that I have deposited. All I had to do was to focus. I needed to understand metabolism, the natural metabolic rate, and how my body burns food for fuel. The body stores its fuel as fat for future use. If you are overweight it could be because of the way you eat, as well as what you eat, and when you eat it.

Boy Scout life's lesson:

I was eleven years old when I went on our first camping trip and learned the importance of building a proper fire with only one match.

Our scout master made it clear that if we wanted to eat, we had to cook the food. In order to cook the food, we had to learn how to make a proper fire. He showed us how to utilize tiny twigs, dry leaves, and plentiful amounts of small kindling. It was much later after the fire was really blazing before we added the larger twigs, broken branches and bigger pieces of wood. Finally, after a hot bed of coals had developed, the fire was large enough to maintain itself. We added the large logs that could burn for hours and still sustain the blaze. It was always a big mistake to put the larger logs on too early for fear that they wouldn't be combustible and burn clear through.

At last, at forty-nine years of age, I finally learned that my body needs to be fed and fueled by the same principles. A fire burns hotter by feeding it smaller kindling often. A fire feeds on energy. A fire burns hotter when smaller amounts of fuel are added more often. The wood burning in the fire is literally the sun's energy that has been stored for years in those twigs, and now the fire is releasing that energy back into the universe in the form of heat and light.

This is also true of your body's metabolism. Your stomach is the furnace used to burn fuel. Your food is the fuel that contains calories and a calorie is a unit of energy. This energy if not used, is converted to fat and stored. All foods have captured the sun's energy and stored it as calories. Vegetables, proteins, breads, oils, fats and all of the food in your pantry is there because of the sun. When eaten, your body converts and metabolizes the food. The body then releases the sun's stored energy in that food for your body to run on. If you feed your body only large meals two or three times a day, it is not going to burn very efficiently, and the excess energy will be stored by the body as fat.

In my late forties, I had spent a year eating sixteen times a day or one hundred calories every hour for sixteen hours. I kept providing my body the kindling in order to feed the fire of my metabolism. In those twelve months I don't ever remember being hungry, or ever exercising. I still lost forty pounds by eating, because my body burned the fat with my natural metabolic rate. Then came the life changing event that would transform my health. It was only two months before my fiftieth birthday when I suffered a heart attack and lived to tell the tale. I immediately quit my pack-a-day smoking habit and substituted it with eating.

Watch over your heart with all diligence:

On March 7, 2009 I was dealing the card game "Let it Ride" at our local area casino. I felt faint, sweaty and out of breath. Immediately I was escorted to the back room where an emergency medical technician took my vitals and helped stabilize me. The arteries that fed the blood to my heart were plugged up and depriving the muscle of oxygen. I was having a heart attack. Thankfully, my employer provides EMT's for their patrons, employees, and an ambulance service is only five minutes away. The ambulance driver was able to administer nitro that helped open the arteries and increase the blood flow to my heart. Within three hours of the attack, the hospitals' on call heart specialist was able to balloon the two arteries nicknamed the "widow maker." He was able to unplug my clogged arteries using angioplasty and a stint. I was lucky that there was no muscle damage to my heart. If I had been on the way home in my car or perhaps in bed asleep, I doubt that I would be here today to tell the tale.

Three years have passed since my angioplasty and heart stint. In that time I quit smoking. I rarely exercised. I ate whatever I wanted, whenever I wanted, and put on weight. I became inactive and developed a hypo-thyroid. All of these factors contributed to driving down my metabolism and driving up my fat deposits.

I began my experiment of combining a proper way of eating along with a proper exercise routine in February of 2012. I weighed an all time record of 262.4 pounds. My knees hurt, my feet hurt, and I couldn't bend over to pick up a pen off of the floor. I had trouble tying my shoes. I knew I had gotten too fat and could relate to my brother-in-law when he said that he had trouble reaching around to wipe his butt! We had a son's wedding reception in a three months and a family reunion later that summer. I finally made the mental decision, adjusted my focus and attitude and then made the commitment to losing weight and getting back into shape.

75 - 20 - 3.5 - 1.5 percent

I am convinced that almost anything you want to achieve in life, including losing weight and getting into shape is seventy five percent psychological, twenty percent focus and attitude, three and a half percent preparing and one and a half percent effort. Let me explain…

75% psychological – Your will is one of the strongest forces in the universe. Have you heard the term "your mind's eye"? Your mind has to *see,* and your heart has to *believe* before any changes in your life can be allowed to take place. Once you overcome the psychological barriers your mind has created over the years, you can begin to change some bad habits and behaviors for the better. Your life is like a locomotive. When standing still a train requires an enormous amount of energy to begin moving. Once in motion, it can propel itself forward with a minimal amount of effort.

20% focus and attitude – All day long you have to choose to do the right thing. Temptation to stray, cheat or take short cuts will confront you every day. Your attitude helps determine your altitude and allow you to soar to unlimited heights of energy and creativity.

3.5% preparing – I spend about six hours a week shopping, cooking, preparing and packaging my meals. 6 divided by 168 = .0357

1.5% effort – I spend ½ hour per day working out for five days. Out of every 168 hours per week I spend 2.5 hours in the gym. 2.5 divided by 168 = .01488

I love food!

I love to eat and I hate being hungry. I despise the word "diet," because in my mind it implies that I have to sacrifice my love of eating. Diets have never worked for me. I was always hungry and constantly thinking of when I could eat next. When I wanted to lose weight the first of every year, I was convinced that I needed to fast, and live on a very low calorie diet. I was inadvertently slowing down my metabolism. My body sensed that food was in short supply and in order to survive it had to store fat for leaner times. Sweets, cookies and sugar treats such as candy bars were almost impossible to say no to. In one sitting I could devour an entire package of oatmeal cookies with two glasses of milk and still be hungry. Chocolate in any form was what I craved and I made sure that it was stashed in the freezer, cabinets and pantry. I became lethargic, tired and any physical activity was easily discouraged. All of these combined behaviors told my body to store the fat, and store the fat it did! I needed to wake my body up and correct some very destructive habits that I had developed. I had no clue that everything I was doing was inadvertently and deliberately slowing down my body's metabolic rate and instructing my body to store energy.

It wasn't until my annual physical at fifty-two, when blood tests revealed to my doctor that I had a hypo-thyroid. My thyroid was under producing a hormone that also helped cause weight gain. I hate taking medication of any kind. I told my doctor that I haven't used drugs in thirty years and I'm not going to start now. Even after my heart condition, I only take a cholesterol medication, a hormone for my thyroid, a baby aspirin for blood thinning, a multi-vitamin, and omega-3s. I was determined to try to learn what I could do to avoid taking any new prescription medication. It was then that I learned that my thyroid should produce a hormone that speeds up my metabolism. Because it was under-active, it was actually slowing down my metabolic rate.

A slow metabolism causes the body to store fat. The slower the metabolic rate in people, the greater the weight gains. Slow metabolism can be caused by several factors. Most factors are a very low calorie diet, fasting, snacking on high sugared foods such as soda pop, candy bars, and gum. Other factors include low physical activity and an under-active thyroid. Little did I realize, I was hitting on all cylinders and doing all the wrong things at once!

One of the biggest challenges I face is to try to understand the differences between my wife's body mass index and her metabolic chemical reactions. There is a definite difference between the two of us as to the caloric needs based on our muscle mass and how our bodies burn fat differently. It seems that I can lose fat faster than she can, and I don't know exactly why. The other challenge I have is trying to help her overcome a psychological barrier. Her subconscious doesn't believe that she can eat food more often and still lose weight. Everything she has been taught in magazines, literature and society is that a woman is not supposed to eat calories. In her mind, calories consumed equals more fat. How can she possibly eat all day long without gaining more weight?

Change your metabolism.

They key to changing your weight is to change your metabolism.

The definition of metabolic activity…

> *Life-sustaining chemical activity. The series of processes by which food is converted into the energy and products needed to sustain life; and, chemical activity involving particular substances. The biochemical activity of a particular substance in a living organism.*

Metabolism can be compared to a vehicle, and described as the speed at which our body's motor is running or the revolutions per minute (RPMs). The higher the RPMs, the more energy it takes to propel the car and keep it in motion. Metabolism is based on the number of calories we need to burn during the day to work, sleep and exist. It is the key to understanding your body and how to burn the fuel it needs. You have to learn to look at food as fuel. The food we eat is the fuel we need. How we eat, how much we eat, when we eat and the type of food we eat, determines how fast and efficient our body runs.

If you want your vehicle to go faster you feed it more fuel. You don't have to be a mechanic and know the intricacies of a motor to know how a combustion engine works. It takes more fuel to drive 75 mph vs. 55 mph or 35 mph. Even teenagers know that if you want to drag main, you need to keep plenty of gas in the tank. If you are the adult paying for the gas, oil and repairs, it will cost you less money when you know how to get the most efficiency out of your fuel. It costs less when you know how to properly maintain your vehicle to avoid costly repairs and break downs. There is not much philosophical difference between the car you drive and the body you maintain. Both require fuel to get you where you want to go, and properly maintained they should last you a long time. How you get to where you want to go, and how much it will cost is completely up to you.

There are two fundamental keys to changing your metabolism:

1. Eat smaller portions and eat more often.

2. Stimulate your heart rate for at least twenty minutes.

As I said earlier, the key to change your weight is to change your metabolism via eating and heart rate. There are two simple ways to help increase your metabolic rate and burn the fat to supply the energy your body has to have in order to sustain your daily activities and life.

Please note, I am not a nutritionist and will not try to educate people on the nutritional balances and proper percentages of proteins, good carbohydrates, bad carbohydrates, good fats, bad fats, and calorie contents of all the combinations of foods you choose to eat. I do, however, believe in some very simple common sense guides to choosing what to eat and choosing what to avoid.

Everyone needs to eat right, and exercise properly. Our population is evidence that we are losing the battle. Weight loss is a zero sum game. By that, I mean you have to burn more calories than you take in. How you burn those calories and how hot you burn them is the key. Allowing your body to do the work is critical.

Here is what I have found to be the easiest path to weight loss and a healthy lifestyle. The simple rule to follow is when at the grocery store buy the food on the perimeter of the store, not on the inside shelves. If you think about it, all the fresh food is around the outer walls. All of the processed foods are on the inside isles of the store. Eat foods that can spoil in one to two weeks, and try to avoid eating processed food. Just remember, it is your choice. You choose your own fate and destiny every day with the decisions you make. My only advice is to choose wisely, and keep it simple.

Dieting now means to eat as often as you can!

I want you to stay focused on changing your metabolism. You can now use food to increase your metabolic activity and burn more fat if done properly with a few easy tools.

The term diet has seemed to always carry a negative connotation. If I was on a diet, it meant that I had to do without food. My diet now means to me that it is the manner in which I eat. I am not dieting and depriving myself of food in order to lose weight. I use my eating habits to fuel increased metabolism. Our stomachs are furnaces used to burn energy. A fire burns hotter and faster if you add small amounts of kindling very often. A fire doesn't burn energy very well if you try to use large logs on a small fire. We are in the habit and have conditioned ourselves to eat breakfast, lunch and dinner every day. We consume three square meals a day, while we throw large logs on a small fire and wonder why it doesn't burn the energy. We snack on high sugared treats, drinks and lots of carbohydrates and wonder why our population is getting so obese. It is no wonder the diet and exercise industry booms after the holidays into spring and summer. Break away from traditions and think outside of the box.

If you are eating all of the time, your body instinctively knows that food is plentiful and will naturally shed the fat it has stored for leaner times. You can trick the body into believing that it doesn't have to store fat if the stomach is constantly digesting and working to absorb its nutrition.

Change your eating habits for five days:

The goal is to consume around 1600-1800 calories per day (depending on whether you are a male or female) and eat as often as possible. Break your food down into 100 calorie portions of proteins, carbohydrates and fats utilizing re-sealable sandwich bags to store and transport your food. During any given day, I try to eat more protein than carbohydrates and fats. I try to eat around fifty percent proteins, forty percent healthy carbohydrates and ten percent healthy fats. There has been a lot of misunderstanding about low carbohydrate and low fat diets. The bottom line is that everything is good in moderation and to keep a balanced outlook on eating fresh foods. Stay away from processed foods when you can.

If I eat every hour, I prefer to alternate between eating proteins one hour, and then healthy carbohydrates the next hour. Examples of healthy carbohydrates are bananas, potatoes, carrots, V8 juice, grapes, fruits and vegetables. Stay away from processed carbohydrates. Carbohydrates provide the energy your body needs and the proteins provide the satiety that will fill you up. If you eat too many carbohydrates too often your body burns them off and will leave you still hungry. If you eat too many proteins too often you may run short of energy and you will end up being tired and lethargic.

If I eat every two hours then I want to eat a protein and a complex carbohydrate to give me an even amount of energy and satiate my appetite. The added benefits are that your blood sugar should remain steady, your concentration and mood level won't be subject to swings when you eat small portions often. Healthy fats are important also.

There are many options that you can adapt to your eating patterns depending on your work environment, personal schedule, and daily obligations. All leading dietitians recommend eating at least five times a day. The solution is to look at your food preparation and food consumption in a completely different light.

Easy five day food preparation:

I make my entire menu for the five work days with one hour of shopping and three hours of food preparation. Then all I have to do each day it to pack up the individual baggies from the fridge and stash them in my cooler on the way to work.

The first thing I did was to substitute my processed loaf of bread for Joseph's Pita Bread. The pita is oat bran and stone ground wheat with no trans-fat and no cholesterol. It has only ten grams of total carbohydrates, five grams of fiber, therefore, only five net grams of carbohydrates per pita. I use the pita bread to spread peanut butter on, or honey nut crème cheese spread, or my famous rice, refried bean, garlic and sausage mixture. This is a great recipe I developed.

I boil one cup of rice, then add a can of refried beans and one pound of cooked, drained sausage or hamburger, with two cloves of pressed garlic. One cup makes a power packed protein and carbohydrate snack that I mix with salsa and blue tortilla chips. Sometimes I will spread it on pita bread for a meal, or just heat and eat by itself. This recipe will make at least ten servings for the week.

I prefer to eat my favorite foods and tailor my eating accordingly. For my carbohydrates, every week I buy five bananas; five cans of V8 juice; one small package of baby carrots that makes five portions; approximately two pounds of grapes, to make five individual portions; five small potatoes and an assortment of fruits such as nectarines, peaches or plums.

For my proteins, I buy one package of sliced cheese and one dozen eggs to hard boil. Five of the eggs I use to eat individually with a slice of cheese, and the rest I make into deviled egg snacks. I buy one package of boneless chicken thighs, (or chicken breasts if you prefer) for grilling five portions. I will purchase one pound of sliced meat of either ham, turkey or beef. Three slices of thinly sliced meat makes one serving. I will also use one cup of cottage cheese on ½ of a baked potato for a serving of carbohydrates and protein.

The main sources for my healthy fats are either a peanut butter pita in the morning, or perhaps ten black olives, ½ an avocado, a handful of nuts or cashews, or my honey nut crème cheese on pita-bread.

Several ways to eat:

People think it is difficult to eat at work, yet how many of you have access to a candy bar, potato chip dispenser or pop machine? People snack at work all the time! It's just that they have conditioned themselves to eat sweets. You can do this if you put your mind to it and change some behaviors and habits.

You could do as I first did for a year and eat 100 calories of food once an hour for sixteen hours. You would be eating sixteen times a day and fueling the fire of your body's metabolism with a lot of little kindling. This can be inconvenient for most people because they need to be able to carry a cooler with them all day long.

If you want, you could eat 200 calories of food once every two hours for sixteen hours and eat eight times a day. I've adapted this habit most recently and have found it very accommodating and easy to do.

Finally, you could eat 300 calories of food every three hours for fifteen hours and eat five times a day, and still have a few snacks in between meals.

My wife doesn't care for my method of eating. She prefers to drink 300 calorie protein drinks twice a day with healthy snacks in between and a healthy dinner in the evening.

I carry a small cooler to work every day filled with individual portions equaling approximately one thousand calories for the eight hours of work and allowing for the commute time back and forth. One hardboiled egg with a slice of cheese, three thinly sliced pieces of meat, one grilled piece of chicken, four ounces of steak, twenty baby carrots, twenty grapes or a choice of fruit, one can of V8 juice, a banana, and my favorite snack of the day; a pita spread with honey nut crème cheese. These are ten 100 calorie portions of proteins, carbohydrates, vegetables and healthy fats while keeping the food groups in pretty good balance.

100 calorie portions: (of my personal favorite foods)

Proteins: Approximate calories

1 hardboiled egg	=	55
1 slice of cheese	=	60
1 1/2 deviled eggs	=	90
1/2 cup cottage cheese	=	100
3 slices of deli ham, turkey or beef	=	100
½ chicken breast	=	100
4 oz steak	=	100
Protein Shakes-(skim milk)	=	200

Carbohydrates:

Joseph's Pita Bread	=	60
1 Tbsp Peanut Butter	=	95
1 can of V8 juice	=	70
1 banana	=	105
20 grapes	=	72
20 baby carrots	=	95
1 potato	=	110
½ potato, ¼ cup cottage cheese	=	100
1 nectarine	=	67
1 apple	=	81

Healthy Fats: (fats are very important!)

2 Tbsp Crème Cheese	=	80
1 Tbsp Peanut Butter	=	95
½ Avocado	=	160
1 tsp Olive Oil	=	40
1 tsp Butter	=	110
10 Black Olives	=	50
1 handful of Cashews	=	100

Burn the fat faster:

Once my mind accepted that the true definition of the word "diet" simply meant a "new way of eating", it was easy to adapt to. I had already spent a year eating every hour on the hour, and my body shed the pounds naturally. This time when I made the decision to lose fifty pounds, I didn't want to have to wait a year just by only eating right. I needed to accelerate the process. I was going to have to do what I despised doing. I was going to have to work out. I realized that I had to incorporate exercise into my weekly schedule. I hate traditional home work out programs or gym memberships as much as I hate dieting. I knew I had a real psychological problem to overcome if I wanted to attain my goal of losing fifty pounds in six months.

When I first adopted this habit of eating for energy, I was in direct home sales. It was my job to help homeowners buy replacement windows and siding for their homes. It was very simple and convenient to carry my food in a cooler and eat every hour. I could even set my watch alarm to alert me every sixty minutes.

Now, I am working in an environment of dual responsibilities. When I work as a dealer on a blackjack table, I get a break every hour and twenty minutes. It allows me to eat 200 calories during every break when dealing. As a dual rate supervisor, or "pit boss", I get a break every two and a half hours. I eat three bags of food or 300 calories every break, and I get three breaks every evening. I have a bag of carrots on my way to work. I treat myself to a pita covered with honey nut crème cheese on the way home. The crème cheese pita is the last of the fuel I eat for the day. After a good six to seven hour sleep, I wake up with a couple cups of coffee and then head to the gym for my five, five minute workouts.

Don't get RIPPED.

The myth for the masses is that anyone can get ripped in ninety days. All of the infomercials that magically appear every January 2nd after the holidays prove my point. The truth is that most people get ripped in the first five minutes when they order from one of the many infomercials promoting their hard bodies and six pack abs. They emotionally purchase the product, and after the first couple of tough workouts in their living room they give up because the emotion has passed and reality of the hard work and the commitment it will take has set in. The videos then sit on the shelf until they find their way to the thrift store, and the bitter reality of another expensive lesson sets in. Their mind is further conditioned to tell them that losing weight just can't be done, and there is no need to try again.

I don't want a ripped body like I had as a wrestler in high school. Those days are long gone. I don't want to build my arm, chest and abdominal muscles. My fifty-two year old body wanted reality and results that were achievable. I instinctively knew that I wanted my natural metabolism back that I had as a young man. I never dreamed that it was my actions and behavior that was causing my metabolic rate to slowly slip away and how I was training my body to deliberately slow its own metabolism and prevent it from burning fat for fuel.

Ever since high school football and wrestling conditioning, I've always disliked working out because it was hard. It took work, discipline and a determination to willingly inflict pain upon my body. I don't like pain. I avoid pain. As far as I am concerned, it takes a real masochist to willingly inflict pain on themselves.

Exercise:

At my age I need low to zero impact exercises in order to go easy on my joints. The cartilage in my knees, ankles, hips and joints is not the same as it was twenty years ago as a young man. I look for low impact, cardio exercises to increase fuel burning efficiency and amplify my metabolic rate. The key to a good cardio workout at my age is to maintain my heart rate between 120-140 beats per minute for at least twenty minutes to maintain good heart health and burn off the calories.

I hate paying for a memberships and dues. Yet I am a firm believer that if it is going to cost me something, I will be determined to get my value out of the expense. I broke down and joined the local YMCA. It costs me $1.40 per day to rent their equipment and their facility. They have all of the resources in a facility that anyone could need. Available is a walking track, a weight room filled with free weights, several treadmills, stair steppers, elliptical riders, bike machines, basketball court, racquetball court, swimming pool, hot tub, showers and a secure locker facility.

The first day in the gym I walked on the treadmill for twenty minutes. I rode the bike for the next twenty minutes and I walked the track for the final twenty minutes. I thought I really needed an hour workout to do any good. I was sore, tired, bored, and I didn't like the pain and discomfort that the hour provided. The memories of all the past failures of previous workouts came flooding back and my mind wanted to tell me that I would never be able to stick to it.

I knew I needed a simple, relatively painless plan that allowed me to achieve the heart rate I needed. I remembered the heart rehab therapy and the six-week program I had to do after my heart attack. I experimented in the gym on the second day of my new workout schedule. The first hour of the first day at the Y discouraged me, so I modified my work out so that I all I had to do was to focus on a single, specific exercise for only five minutes at a time. This seemed to inflict minimal pain. Since I developed my five minute workout, I actually look forward to my half hour and am disappointed if I miss a day to rest. It has become easy to let my body do the work and naturally fuel my metabolic rate and burn the fat for the fuel it needs.

The five minute workout:

Aka: The two song, five minute, 15 second burn, 5 day workout. All you need is a headset with AM/FM tuner, a bottle of water, green tea, or Gatorade, and thirty minutes of your time per day for five days. I choose to exercise on the days I work so as to have a full two days off to rest and relax.

Many consultants advise exercising at the end of the day before dinner when your metabolism is on the decline. With my schedule it is difficult to work out at five in the morning after my swing shift at work. Therefore, I try to make sure I get my five-minute workout just after I wake up from a six to seven hour sleep. After my morning coffee, I put on my gym clothes and head for the Y with a bottle of flavored water and a radio headset to listen with. I haven't eaten, so my body is running on residual energy from the day before. I personally believe that my body will burn the fat quicker on an empty stomach with plenty of fluids to flush my system with.

The key to changing your metabolism is not to concentrate on how many calories you burn. The key is that you want to get to your target heart rate (*THR*) as soon as possible and maintain it for at least the next twenty minutes. I call this the five-minute workout because you are only going to utilize one cardio machine at a time for five minutes. As soon as the five minutes is over, you move over to the next machine and work on a different set of muscles. Five minutes is not a long time to stay focused and exert your best effort. You are using a new set of muscles and can watch your progress minute by minute so the time flies by. Any cardio exercise will do with or without machines.

Equipment needed: *(no equipment necessary, only cardio exercises!)*

I prefer to use four different cardio exercise machines that seem to suit me best. Choose machines or exercises that you like so that you enjoy the time spent. I spend only five minutes for each exercise. It is critical that you maintain your target heart rate during each five minute session. As your stamina improves, the better shape your leg muscles become, and over time you will have to push yourself a little harder each week in order to reach and maintain your *THR*.

I have found that having a radio headset is critical. It takes two songs to finish each five minutes. Also, most songs have a beat that you can set your workout pace to and help push you to stay in synchronization with. The music playing, or talk radio host also helps distract from the effort and energy you are exerting to maintain your *THR*.

Diminishing resistance, and increasing marginal returns.

This next point is important for psychological reasons. I call it "the principle of diminishing resistance." Your mind wants to choose the path of least resistance. Therefore, I start each machine with the maximum amount of resistance that is still reasonable. As each minute passes, I decrease the resistance setting. This way, as time passes it gets easier minute by minute. Your mind accepts that the worst is behind you and that it will get easier as time passes. Remember, your goal is maintaining your *THR*, not how many calories you burned or how much muscle you are building.

The first thing I do is to stretch my muscles and spend a few minutes walking the track so that my muscles can loosen up. I try to keep a brisk pace to make it easier to reach my *THR* of 120-140 beats per minute as I begin on the equipment.

The 15 second burn.

The last fifteen seconds on each five minute session needs to be used to really pump up your heart rate. This enables you to effectively move to the next machine, adjust the settings and begin your next session with your *THR* still in the zone. When my time clock reaches 4:45, I maximize the resistance level and give the best effort I can.

1st Five:

The first five minutes I spend on the treadmill. Each treadmill has automated settings that account for time elapsed, distance walked, speed, elevation, and even handles to hold in order to measure your heart rate. I start with the incline at 5% while maintaining 3.5 mph for the first two and a half minutes. I then increase the incline to 10% and maintain the speed at 3.5 mph for the final two and a half minutes. My heart rate has been within my target zone of 120-140 beats per minute. I have effectively worked my calves and am ready to work on my gluts and thighs.

2nd Five:

The next five minutes are spent on the elliptical machine. This is the toughest machine for me personally, so it is one of the first I begin with. In this way, my mind knows that the workout will get easier as time goes on. I increase the resistance to the point it is difficult and makes me strain to push the rotations. I watch for each one minute mark, and each minute that expires, I reduce the resistance by one setting. It doesn't take long to achieve five individual one minute intervals. The final 15 seconds I maximize the resistance level and push myself until I "feel the burn." My heart is pounding, and this allows me time to move to the next machine with my heart rate in the zone.

3rd Five:

The next five minutes I spend on the stair stepper. My goal is to set the resistance high enough to make me work, yet low enough to allow me to reach my goal of 500 stairs in 5 minutes. I have 300 seconds to walk up 500 stairs or 100 stairs every 60 seconds. This is excellent for your thigh muscles. This is the one machine that I don't reduce the resistance on as each minute passes. I have found it difficult to maintain my heart rate if the resistance isn't high enough, so I have to increase my repetitions to make up for any lack of resistance. Again, the final fifteen seconds is important to increase the resistance and push yourself to finish strong.

4th Five:

The next five minutes are spent on the bike. Again, the key is to set the resistance high enough to make you sweat and make your heart pound. It always amazes me to watch people spend twenty minutes on a bike with no resistance as they pedal away. Why would they waste their time just to move their legs? Work your legs and make it as intense as you can for only five minutes, you'll be glad you did. In the final fifteen seconds you need to pedal hard and maximize your effort. You can sure tell you are in the zone when your heart is pounding and the sweat is flowing! I always carry a bottle of flavored water to keep hydrated.

Final Five:

Finally, I spend the last five minutes back on the treadmill where I began. I set the speed at a full 4.0 miles per hour and the incline at 15%. The final five minutes I push myself to finish strong with a solid effort. The closer to the five minute mark I get, the more I will decrease the incline and decrease the speed so that it gets easier as the time passes.

Cool down:

I use the basketball court, or the walking track to walk and cool down for the last few minutes. The cool down period is important to allow your body to re-acclimate itself and let the muscles rest.

Recharge electrolytes and nutrients lost:

Proper after-work out nutrition is very important. You need to replenish the vitamins, proteins, simple and complex carbohydrates that you just used up. I found the orange flavored P90X Results and Recovery Formula is an excellent source of everything I need.

Hydration:

Keep the fluids flowing! Plenty of water in your system allows the cells in your body to dispose of the waste products more effectively and flush your system. Drinking water for me is boring. I need flavored water to satisfy my drinking needs. I used to buy Lipton's green tea until I found their packets of Lipton's "Revitalize" raspberry lime iced tea mix. I can buy ten packets for a dollar and only spend ten cents per sixteen ounce bottle instead of fifty cents per bottle for the premade convenient brands. The added benefit is that each serving has zero calories and daily servings equal to 50% Vitamin C, 25% Vitamin B6, 25% Vitamin B12, and 20% Niacin. Now that I found what I really like, I drink them all day long.

Plateau: *To reach a level, period or condition of stability*

If you are tracking your weight in order to measure your progress I highly recommend weighing yourself only once a week. One reason is that as your body starts burning fat for energy it is also increasing muscle in your legs. Muscle weighs more than fat, and there may come a time where your weight doesn't change much. You could become discouraged if it is only weight loss that you are trying to measure. The key is to stay consistent, stay focused and strive to meet your daily goals. Each day that you accomplish your goal is one more step toward your final destination.

Results:

One half hour a day is all it is taking me to transform my life. During and after my workout I make sure to drink a lot of fluid. This helps to keep me hydrated, and it reduces my appetite. It is usually an hour or two after my workout that my appetite returns. I begin by eating protein so that by body burns the fat reserves and I can easily begin eating all day for the rest of the day.

Within the first two weeks of eating properly and spending thirty minutes a day exercising, I discovered endorphins and the natural euphoria that accompanies a good workout. It is a fantastic natural high! My body is being fueled by an appropriate way of eating. I am consuming proper nutrients, appropriate vitamins, drinking correct fluids while obtaining the necessary exercise for my heart health. I am sleeping a solid six hours and waking up refreshed. It has been a long time since I felt this good while growing older. On my two days off of exercise, I eat regular healthy meals with proper snacks in between so as to maintain my metabolic rate.

Two days off:

Take a break. This doesn't mean to quit practicing good eating habits. It means that everyone needs a break from the grind and the same ol' same ol'. Taking a break does not mean falling back into bad habits and routines. I still enjoy eating three regular meals a day. However, I have learned, thanks to Dr. Oz and his TV show, how to eat healthy snacks one to two hours before meals. Healthy snacks combined with a few diet aids with meals can really help the body's metabolism and curb the cravings we all have. I want to share the information Dr. Oz shared on his show pertaining to healthy snacks and natural diet aids.

Healthy snacks:

These recipes are approximately 200 calories each. They are a pre-dinner snack you should eat one to two hours before dinner. They each have approximately six grams of fiber to kick start the digestive process, and ten grams of protein that help turn on hormones to burn fat and satiate your appetite. These help speed up your metabolism and also keep you from overeating at dinner.

> *Cheese Wrap:*
> > *Thin slice of smoked turkey or ham*
> > *wrapped around 2% string cheese*
> > *2 green olives*
> > *1 cup zucchini*
> > *¼ cup chickpeas*

> *Mini Pizza Pocket:*
> > *1 mini whole wheat pita pocket*
> > *1 oz 2% reduced fat mozzarella cheese*
> > *2 TBSP pasta sauce – 1 cup spinach – 2 onion slices*

> *Chips and Dip:*
> > *½ cup 2% Greek Yogurt*
> > *1 tsp walnuts*
> > *garlic– black pepper*
> > *1 tsp hot sauce, 1 cup cherry tomatoes*
> > *1 1/2 oz blue tortilla chips* (important)*

Cheesy Apple Sandwich:
- *4 apple slices*
- *3 TBSP low fat ricotta cheese*
- *10 almonds*
- *Lemon juice*

Pizza Popcorn:
- *High Volume – Low Calorie Snack*
- *3 TBSP popcorn kernels = 8 cups of popped popcorn*
- *1 TBSP garlic powder*
- *1 TBSP paprika*
- *1 TBSP oregano*
- *1 tsp salt – 1 tsp chives*

Peanut Butter Quesadilla:
- *Mid Morning – Late Afternoon Snack*
- *Mini whole wheat tortilla*
- *¼ cup banana slices (five slices)*
- *1 TBSP peanut butter*
- *A pinch of cinnamon*

Onion Rings:
- *To curb salt craving*
- *Slice an Onion*
- *1 egg*
- *1 tsp oregano*
- *¼ tsp Old Bay Spice*
- *Bake at 350° in oven 20-30 minutes*

No Bake Chewy Chocolate Truffles
- *To curb sweet cravings*
- *5 dried dates*
- *11 dried apricots*
- *¼ cup raw cocoa powder*
- *½ TBSP vanilla extract (stick coconut together)*
- *1 TBSP agave nectar (stick nuts together)*
- *½ cup unsweetened coconut*
- *½ cup chopped hazelnut and pinch of salt*

Natural diet aids with meals:

These help curb appetite, increase metabolism and aid digestion;

> *Morning Breakfast:*
> *Sage Leaf Tea with the meal*

> *Lunch:*
> *Alpha Lipoic Acid**
> *Maitake Mushroom Extract* 20 drops in a glass of water*
> *This controls cravings without the dip in sugar levels.*

> *Dinner:*
> *Glucomannen**
>> *Powerful fiber – mix with a small glass of water*
>> *½ hour before your meal, and after your snack.*

*Consult your physician before using these over the counter products.

Dessert: ***What would life be without a treat!***
(1 cup = 150 calories)

> *5 layer Cake:*
>> *1ˢᵗ Layer:*
>>> *Dark chocolate cake mix*
>>> *1 cup greek yogurt*
>>> *1 cup water*
>>> *Mix ingredients*
>>> *Bake in cake pan @ 350°*
>> *2ⁿᵈ Layer:*
>>> *4 cups Ricotta*
>>> *1 cup coconut milk*
>>> *1 cup shredded toasted coconut*
>>> *4 TBSP Agave Syrup*
>> *3ʳᵈ Layer:*
>>> *½ cup toasted oats*
>>> *½ cup ground flax seed*
>>> *½ cup fine chopped walnuts*
>>> *Shake in a bag – spread on top*

4th *Layer:*
    Berries: Custom make to taste
    1 cup each;
    Strawberries, Blueberries, Raspberries,
    Blackberries
5th *Layer:*
    Bittersweet chocolate
    Vegetable peeler – use to shred liberally on top

Food allergies:

My wife suffered for years with sinus infections and often would feel tired and lethargic. She couldn't understand why she had no energy and felt bad all of the time. Through medical testing, she found out she had a sensitivity to certain foods. Foods containing gluten (rye, wheat, barley and oats if processed in the same facility as other grains) and dairy products that contain a protein called casein were the culprits. She referred me to the following commentary from an article on the web. (http:/naturalhealthschool.com/foodallergies.html).

According to medical estimates, 60% of Americans suffer from food allergies. Food allergies also referred to as food sensitivities or food reactions, can result in digestive disturbances such as gas, belching and bloating after meals. They can also cause symptoms not related to the digestive system including headaches, migraines, joint pain, arthritis, hyperactivity, skin rashes, asthma, dry cough, wheezing, diarrhea, kidney damage and elevated liver enzymes. Food allergies can make you feel lethargic, sleepy, or low in energy, especially after eating. They can also be responsible for mood swings and cravings.

Food allergies and unexplained weight gain.

The food that you crave are also the foods that you are likely to be allergic to. Some people feel that they are addicted to their problem foods. It is not the food itself but the endorphins – the body's opium-like pain killers which are triggered by the problem foods that they are addicted to. Because of the cravings associated with food allergies, there is a tendency to overeat and weight gain is likely to be a problem. For underweight individuals food allergies may have the opposite effect, making it difficult for them to gain weight. Both overweight and underweight individuals often find it easier to reach and maintain their ideal weight when their food allergies are properly addressed through nutrition and lifestyle changes.

Two kinds of food allergies.

*There are two basic types of food allergies depending on that type of antibodies produced by the body in response to the offending food. The first is what is called **IgE** food allergies that account for only 5% of all adverse food reactions and affect approximately 1 to 2% of the population (ear, nose and throat). These are the allergies that received the most attention from the medical profession because symptoms appear almost immediately – within minutes to a few hours after consuming the food. The symptoms associated with this type of food allergies generally affect the skin (e.g. rash), airways (e.g. asthma), and digestive tract (e.g. gas, belching, bloating, and pain).*

My wife has an immediate reaction to dairy products, some worse than others depending on how they are processed. Sour cream is her worst culprit. Sour cream causes sinus congestion and pain. The only two dairy products that don't affect her are butter and cottage cheese. These two items do not contain the protein casein.

The article states that *the second type of food allergy is the **IgG** type which accounts for 95% of all adverse food reactions and affect nearly 60% of the American population. These frequently go undiagnosed for years because the reactions are delayed or hidden, with onset of symptoms occurring hours to days after the offending food is consumed; and because they present chronic symptoms involving multiple body systems and not just the digestive system. Some doctors will argue that food allergies are uncommon; this is because they are thinking only of the first allergies mentioned earlier. Unfortunately, medical training regarding the more chronic and insidious conditions, such as those brought about by the much more common allergies, leaves much to be desired.*

To learn more about food allergies, my wife suggests that one of the best books written is "Dangerous Grains" by author James Braly. He thoroughly explains how food allergies affect the body and your overall health.

For those of you who have food allergies and those who think this might be the culprit in your lives, don't despair, as there are steps you can take and food that you can eat to put you on the right step to better health. For more information on food allergies, please go to the website listed previously.

My wife now purchases gluten and dairy free products at the local grocery store. She had been looking for a protein shake that was allergen free (gluten and dairy) that is relatively inexpensive to supplement her diet. Through a friend she discovered *Herbalife* (www.herbalife.com). Some of you may be familiar with this product and for those of you who are not; it is a fabulous meal replacement. These shakes consist of about 200+ calories, depending on what you put in them and the type of dairy products used. My wife uses rice or almond milk products. These shakes replace a regular meal, and when combined with healthy snacks, they curb her appetite, reduce her cravings for sweets, and still fires up her metabolism.

She usually has a delicious protein shake for breakfast and lunch. She snacks around ten in the morning and three in the afternoon. She can still have a great meal in the evening and thus she eats five to six times a day. For her exercise she prefers to walk in the evenings with her sister, and work in the yard for her vitamin D.

I have included just a few of the recipes for the shakes with a list of other shakes that are available. Besides the gluten and allergen free vanilla, there are Cookies and Cream, Chocolate, French Vanilla, Pina Colada and Wild Berry. If you can't find a flavor you like among the list of possible selections, then you had better have your taste buds medically tested!

Protein shake recipes: (blender needed)

All shakes have 8 oz of milk or milk substitutes such as rice milk, almond, coconut or soy milk.

Add 8 oz of ice after you blend all the ingredients to make a creamy shake.

Butterscotch
>8 oz of milk or milk substitute
>2 scoops Formula 1 French Vanilla protein powder
>2 TBSP butterscotch pudding dry mix

Blueberry Muffin
>8 oz of milk or milk substitute
>2 scoops of Formula 1 French Vanilla protein powder
>¼ cup of frozen blueberries
>1 TBSP of pistachio pudding dry mix
>1 tsp of Splenda or other sugar substitute

French Vanilla
>8 oz of milk or milk substitute
>2 scoops of Formula 1 French Vanilla protein powder
>½ cap of vanilla extract
>1 TBSP of vanilla pudding dry mix

Cherry Cobbler
>8 oz of milk or milk substitute
>2 scoops of Formula 1 French Vanilla protein powder
>¼ cup of frozen cherries
>1 capful of almond extract
>½ tsp of dry cherry Jell-0 top with crushed graham crackers

How many choices would you like? (Recipes are available from Herbalife)

Vanilla Orange	Vanilla Coffee Shake	Apple Pie
Orange Julius	Dreamsicle	Peach Mango
Vanilla Orange Banana	Cherry Cheesecake	Vanilla Mint
Vanilla Almond	Orange Cream	Apple Pie
Strawberry Banana	Vanilla Cappuccino	Banana Bread
Blueberry Cheesecake	Blueberry Cobbler	Banana Nut
Carmel Apple Pie	Choc Raspberry Cheesecake	Butter Pecan
Pineapple Upside Down	White Chocolate Mint	Mango Pango
Elvis and PB & Banana	Kiwi Quencher	Key Lime Pie
Strawberry Cheesecake	Blueberry Almond Cheesecake	Almond Joy
Banana Crème Pie	Pistachio Shake	Mudslide
French Toast Shake	Peaches'n Cream	Wedding Cake
Lemon Ice Box	Pineapple Orange Coconut	Butterfinger
Elaine's Lemon Cheesecake	Blueberry/Banana Shake	Snickers
Raspberry Fluff	Orange Mango	Tagalong
Rocky Road with Almonds	Rocky Road with Pecans	Cinnabon
Red Velvet Cake	Original Dutch Chocolate	Samoa

Chocolate Banana	German Chocolate Cake	Oreo Shake
Chocolate Almond	Chocolate Mint	Reese's Shake
Chocolate Strawberry	Chocolate Carmel Cheesecake	Hot Chocolate
Chocolate Chunky Monkey	Chocolate Coconut Cream	Pina Colada
Jamoca Almond Fudge	Chocolate Cappuccino	Hawaiian
Black Forest Cherry	Chocolate Coffee	Wild Berry
Chocolate Raspberry	Chocolate Peanut Butter	Fruit Blast
Chocolate Peanut Butter Banana	Chocolate Carmel Cappuccino	Very Berry
Irish Café' Mocha	Chocolate Covered Cherries	Jazzer-berry
Chocolate Cheesecake	Wedding Cake	Tropical fruit
Turtle Cheesecake	Rice Krispy Treat	Cherry Mash
Oatmeal Cookie	Chocolate No Bake Cookie	Coco Loco
Cookies and Crème Vanilla	White Chocolate Reeces	Café Latte
Chocolate Cookies N Crème	White Chocolate Blueberry	Walnut Latte
Banana Cookies N Crème	Nutter Butter Shake	
Nan's Frozen Strawberry	Banana Split Shake	
Strawberry Berry Cheesecake	Aloha Delight	
Pina Coloda/Raspberry with OJ	Strawberry Pina Colada	
Wild Berry Strawberry	Wild Berry Strawberry Splash	
Tropical Fruit Splash	Tropical Fruit Delight	
Wild Berry Orange Surprise	Carmel Café Latte	
Irish Café Latte	Chocolate Macadamia Café Latte	
Raspberry Latte	Strawberry Latte	
Pecan Honey Soy Latte	Blackberry Hazelnut Soy Latte	
Hazelnut Café Latte	Chocolate Mint Café Latte	

Adaptation:

Use these ideas and principles to adapt them to your own individual lifestyle. There is no single solution or one size fits all that will conform to everyone. Every individual has different work schedules, different break times, and a variety of times available on any given day that allows you to eat. It is easy to use your work environment as an excuse not to eat often. Deliberately look for ways to be creative in order to fuel the fire of your natural metabolism. If you are in an office setting, explain your goals and ask permission from your boss to eat small portions all day long. I give examples of my personal eating preferences, but it is up to you to adapt the concepts to foods that you like and incorporating variety into your weekly routine so that stagnation and boredom don't set in.

My wife and I like completely different foods and eating preferences. However, the basic principles remain constant and the substance of the ideas remains intact for each of us to adapt our own individual likes and dislikes.

Goal setting:

I learned long ago how to set goals, make lists, write down affirmations and take small steps to help achieve my dreams (and now my bucket list!). If your goal is to create wealth, a good banker will tell you to get out of debt, spend less and save more. If your goal is to win friends and influence people, a good mother will encourage you to love more, and criticize less. If your goal is to reduce stress, a good spouse will encourage you to travel more and "get busy livin." If your goal is to lose weight and get in shape, a good doctor will advise you to "diet and exercise." All of these examples are good advice that is easy to say, but can be difficult to do. My goal here is to help you in thirty days change bad habits and develop healthy ones. I want you to believe in your heart and know with your mind that your goals can be achieved in order to transform your behavior to make it come true.

Goals need to be written down, and reviewed often. Break each goal down into annual, monthly, weekly and daily commitments. They must be reasonable, achievable and attainable. Otherwise, as soon as you falter, you become discouraged and tell yourself and your mind that it can't be done. Once you believe in your heart and your mind changes its perceptions, your body will follow. It takes three weeks to break a bad habit and develop a new habit to replace it. Make sure you have a monthly goal that you can achieve over a four week period. Success will breed success, and all things will get easier as time passes.

Variation:

Variety is the spice of life. In the same way that spices make your food fun to eat, everyone should use variety to make living fun. Look for ways to change and adapt your routine so that you don't fall into a rut. I have often heard that if you stay in a rut long enough you are eventually looking up and out of a grave.

Walking is the best exercise by far. Walking is low impact, easy on your joints, good for your heart and free of charge! Walking allows you to get fresh air and enjoy the outdoors. If you like to walk you can choose to walk at the mall or gymnasium during inclement weather. You can walk or ride a bike at a cemetery, walking trails around town, and at local high school track stadiums, etc. Look for ways to bring change into your routines and habits, whether in your daily exercises or in the choice of foods and nutrition you eat.

Variety is one of the keys to making sure you keep your focus and attention on your goals. It can really help you maintain the 20% of your effort and keep your concentration on track.

Affirmations:

Affirmations are powerful tools to help change behavior. If you can visualize what you want and combine it with strong emotional feelings, your mind will change your behavior subconsciously. Behavioral scientists believe you can literally speak into existence the things you want to happen in your life. If you can visualize them and believe them in your heart, they will come to pass. "Watch over your heart with all diligence for from it flow the forces of Life" *Prov. 3:4*

When I began my transformation I had my wife take a picture of my full profile with my shirt off. I wanted a beginning, a place to remember just how fat and out of shape I was. Mainly, I wanted a reminder that I never want to be this heavy and out of shape again.

The next step was to put in writing my goals and break them down into very attainable steps that I could achieve. The key is that the goals had to be reasonable, and they had to be obtainable. I wrote down that I wanted to get the weight off of my knees and joints. I set a six month goal of losing fifty pounds in one hundred and eighty days. I wanted to be able to pass a stress test in ninety days. (Just ask a cardiologist or heart patient how difficult a stress test can be) I needed to lose about eight pounds per month or two pounds per week. This broke down to .296 pounds per day, or close to 800 to 1000 calories per day. I wanted to exercise five minutes at a time, a half hour per day five days a week. I wanted two days a week to rest, relax, have fun, eat regular meals and enjoy my time off.

I have since learned the actual math of CICO *(calories in/calories out)*. My wife and I really enjoy the hit show "Big Bang Theory" so if the math works, it must be reality! I digress, here is how the math is applied…the approximate number of calories in a pound of fat is four thousand. Men typically have more muscle than women, therefore require more calories, and can generally lose fat faster. To find out my specific needs at my age, weight, height, I went on the internet to "nutrition.about.com." My body needs about three thousand calories a day to live and maintain its weight. With a half an hour of exercise each day the caloric intake increases to three thousand two hundred and sixty eight calories per day. These numbers are based on a strict calorie in, calorie out basis (CICO). They take into no account the increased metabolism resulting from eating often. Here are the numbers and the math to calculate how much time was needed to meet my goals.

$$
\begin{array}{ll}
& 3{,}000 \text{ calories to maintain weight without exercise} \\
- & \underline{1{,}800} \text{ calories intake per day for food and nutrition} \\
= & 1{,}200 \text{ calories per day to burn fat for energy}
\end{array}
$$

4,000 calories per pound of fat
50 lbs of fat x 4,000/ lb = 200,000 total calories to burn
200,000 calories / 1,200 per day = 166 days
166 days / 30 days per month = 5.5 months total time

The questions that I needed answered for my goals were?

1. Is this reasonable?
2. Is this achievable?
3. Is this attainable?
4. Can I comfortably limit myself to 1,800 calories a day without feeling like I am dieting or depriving myself?
5. How much pain is going to be involved to achieve this?

Next, I taped the picture of my "fat self", with a print out of my goals on my bathroom mirror. This way, every day in the bathroom I can visualize where I started from and see what I have to do that day to make it happen.

Here is the copy of the goals I wrote down and I keep in front of me every day to help maintain my focus and determination. I have also included a copy of my personal "Bucket List" of long term goals.

My Goals for weight loss:

Lose 50 lbs. in 180 days
8.3 lbs per month
2.07 lbs per week
.296 lbs per day
Weigh 210 lbs. by August 1st.
Pass a stress test by May 1st
Consume 1,800 calories per day
Burn 1000 – 1,200 calories per day
Exercise five days a week at the YMCA
Get the weight off of my knees and joints
Exercise ½ hour per day in 5 minute intervals at a time
Eat 5 to 7 times a day or more

My Bucket List:

Fishing trip to Canada
Scuba dive the Great Barrier Reef
Tour the northeast U.S. in the autumn
Bunge jump over the ravine at Royal Gorge
Skydive – Jump out of a perfectly good airplane

Visit with my wife:

> Niagara Falls
> Valley Forge
> Washington D.C.
> Smokey Mountains
> Tour Europe by car
> Smithsonian Institute
> New York Broadway Show
> Redwood Forest in California
> Banif National Park in Canada
> Glacier National Park in Montana
> Yosemite National Park in California

Most of these goals are very reasonable, achievable and attainable. I intend to cross them off of my list one by one until they are memories.

Conclusion:

Albert Einstein said it best. "The definition of insanity is doing the same thing over and over expecting different results." If you keep doing what you have been doing, you will keep getting what you have been getting. Why would you expect anything else? Be honest with yourself. Look yourself in the mirror just like I did and search out why you failed at every other diet and exercise program you have ever tried? Is it because it was too hard and too boring to maintain? Your mind has conditioned itself to choose the path of least resistance and you have forgotten how good it feels to be in shape. Please trust me when I tell you that this is the easiest adjustment to my lifestyle that I have ever done. I stayed focused for twenty one days (three weeks) and I created altogether new habits. If you choose to modify some behaviors and give it three weeks to change some bad habits, what have you got to lose? I want to encourage you to try something different. Make a difference in your life and then maybe you can be a catalyst to help change the lives of others.

You now have your time invested in reading my pontifications and allowing me to elaborate on the few nuggets of truth that I have learned over the years. If this little booklet has helped you, I want to ask you to help someone else and pay it forward. Give this booklet to someone else who may want to indulge themselves.

I firmly believe life's basic principle that what goes around, comes around and what you sow is what you reap. Please help sow some positive seeds into the fertile soil of the hearts of the people you love.

Thank you for your investment of time and energy.

Sincerely,
Josey Klearley

Be an Optimist:

I strongly urge everyone to get involved in a service organization. Give of yourself and some of your time to your local community. My wife and I have enjoyed our time with the Southwest Optimist Club here in Kansas. If you are looking for a reason to get involved please look for a local chapter in your area.

THE OPTIMIST CREED

Promise yourself

To be so strong that nothing can disturb your peace of mind.

To talk health, happiness, and prosperity to every person you meet.

To make all your friends feel that there is something in them.

To look at the sunny side of everything and make your optimism come true.

To think only of the best, to work only for the best, and to expect only the best.

To be just as enthusiastic about the success of others as you are about your own.

To forget the mistakes of the past and press on to the greater achievements of the future.

To wear a cheerful countenance at all times and give every living creature a smile.

To give so much time to the improvement of yourself that you have no time to criticize others.

To be too large for worry, too noble for anger, too strong for fear, and too happy to permit the presence of trouble.

In loving memory of my Maternal Grandmother

Maud Chamberlin

DESIDERATA

GO PLACIDLY AMID THE NOISE & HASTE, & REMEMBER
WHAT PEACE THERE MAY BE IN SILENCE. AS FAR AS
POSSIBLE WITHOUT SURRENDER BE ON GOOD TERMS
WITH ALL PERSONS. *Speak your truth quietly & clearly; and
listen to others, even the dull & ignorant; they too have their story.
Avoid loud & aggressive persons; they are vexations to the spirit. If
you compare yourself with others, you may become vain & bitter;
for always there will be greater & lesser persons than yourself.
Enjoy your achievements as well as your plans. Keep interested in
your own career, however humble; it is a real possession in the
changing fortunes of time. Exercise caution in your business
affairs; for the world is full of trickery. But let this not blind you to
what virtue there is; many persons strive for high ideals; and
everywhere life is full of heroism. Be yourself. Especially, do not
feign affection. Neither be cynical about love; for in the face of all
aridity & disenchantment it is as perennial as the grass. Take kindly
the counsel of the years, gracefully surrendering the things of youth.
Nurture strength of spirit to shield you in sudden misfortune. But
do not distress yourself with imaginings. Many fears are born of
fatigue & loneliness. Beyond a wholesome discipline, be gentle with
yourself. You are a child of the universe, no less than the trees or
the stars; you have a right to be here. And whether or not it is clear
to you, no doubt the universe is unfolding as it should. Therefore be
at peace with God, whatever you conceive Him to be, and whatever
your labors & aspirations, in the noisy confusion of life keep peace
with your soul. With all its sham, drudgery & broken dreams, it is
still a beautiful world. Be careful. Strive to be happy.*
Max Ehrmann 1927

One Hundred Calorie Appetite
Combined
With The
 Five Minute Workout
Eat all day, every day.
Work out in five minute increments.
Never be hungry and feel the fat melt away.

I lost thirty pounds in ninety days by eating! I have never accomplished something so easily once I set my mind to achieve my goals.

100 calorie appetite combined with the 5 minute workout is a philosophical and psychological approach to common sense eating and exercising. You will learn to treat food as the source of energy your body needs to operate, and understand how your metabolic activity works. Once you fire up your metabolism using proper eating techniques, fresh food, and easy to follow five minute cardio exercises for heart health, you will feel the fat melt away.

All of my life I have hated working out, walking, bike riding, or any type of deliberate routine exercises. Once I started working out in five minute increments, I overcame the mental preconceptions, psychological walls and barriers that I had built into my psyche over the years.

Now that my natural endorphins have kicked in, I have more natural energy and physical drive than I've had since my twenties. I haven't felt this young in so many years! I wish I had known then what I know now!

I feel that I was able to take my mother and father's philosophical outlook and compliment it with my belief in the spiritual reality of God's love. What began as a journal of mine, ended in a booklet designed to help people.
I hope it does as much or more for you as it has done for me.

Josey Klearley

To Order Booklets:

Please visit *dancingwithlightning.com*